Keto Bread

Low-Carb Bakers Recipes for Keto Buns, Bagels, Muffins, Flatbread, Tortillas, Cornbread, Loaves and more

Faith Smith

About The Author

For most of my life, I did not have to worry too much about my weight; I was not the fittest person but I was also not overweight, which was good enough for me. However, after I gave birth to my lovely son, things changed; I gained quite a bit of weight and I did not exactly like what I saw. I was not as confident as I once was and I was very conscious of how I looked and how the clothes I wore made me look. Once my son turned one and was not breastfeeding as much, I started researching for ways to lose weight.

In my quest to lose weight, I have tried quite a bit of different things from the ketogenic diet and intermittent fasting to smoothie cleanses. Since all these have worked for me, I have incorporated them into my lifestyle and I must say, so far I like what I see.

I understand how difficult losing weight can be and to make it easier for you, I write books on what has worked for me and how you can lose weight to achieve your desired body.

I have still not achieved my dream body but I am happy with the progress so far and that is good enough because life is not perfect and I am okay with good enough.

Keto Bread

© Copyright 2019 by Faith Smith - All rights reserved.

This document is geared towards providing exact and reliable information in regards to the topic and issue covered. The publication is sold with the idea that the publisher is not required to render accounting, officially permitted, or otherwise, qualified services. If advice is necessary, legal or professional, a practiced individual in the profession should be ordered.

- From a Declaration of Principles which was accepted and approved equally by a Committee of the American Bar Association and a Committee of Publishers and Associations.

In no way is it legal to reproduce, duplicate, or transmit any part of this document in either electronic means or in printed format. Recording of this publication is strictly prohibited and any storage of this document is not allowed unless with written permission from the publisher. All rights reserved.

The information provided herein is stated to be truthful and consistent, in that any liability, in terms of inattention or otherwise, by any usage or abuse of any policies, processes, or directions contained within is the solitary and utter responsibility of the recipient reader. Under no circumstances will any legal responsibility or blame be held against the publisher for any reparation, damages, or monetary loss due to the information herein, either directly or indirectly.

Respective authors own all copyrights not held by the publisher.

The information herein is offered for informational purposes solely, and is universal as so. The presentation of the information is without contract or any type of guarantee assurance.

The trademarks that are used are without any consent, and the publication of the trademark is without permission or backing by the trademark owner. All trademarks and brands within this book are for clarifying purposes only and are the owned by the owners themselves, not affiliated with this document.

Table of Contents

About The Author — 2

Introduction — 8

Chapter 1: Keto Buns and Bagels — 9

    Keto Buns — 9

    Almond Flour Buns — 11

    Tasty Keto Buns — 13

    Fluffy Buns — 16

    Cheesy Hamburger Buns — 18

    Ultimate Keto Buns — 20

    Keto Bagels — 22

    Rosemary Bagels — 24

    Keto Bagel — 26

    Mozzarella Dough Bagels — 28

Chapter 2: Keto Muffins — 30

    Walnut Flax Muffins — 30

    Peanut Butter Muffins — 32

    Chocolate Zucchini Muffins — 34

    Keto Chocolate Muffins — 36

    Blackberry-Filled Keto Muffins — 38

Coffee Cake Muffins _____ 41

Keto Blueberry Muffins _____ 44

Chapter 3: Keto Loaves _____ 46

Fluffy Keto Bread Loaf _____ 46

Dairy Free Keto Loaf_____ 48

Simple Almond Flour Bread_____ 50

Keto Bread _____ 52

Best Keto Bread _____ 54

Sesame Seed Keto Bread _____ 56

Low Carb Bread _____ 58

Chapter 4: Keto "Cornbread" Recipes_____ 61

Keto "Cornbread"_____ 67

Low Carb Cornbread_____ 69

Almond Flour "Cornbread" _____ 71

Tasty Keto Cornbread _____ 74

Simple Keto Cornbread _____ 76

Chapter 5: Keto Flatbread and Tortilla Recipes _____ 78

Keto Flatbread_____ 78

Indian Flatbread _____ 80

Low-Carb Flatbread _____ 82

5-ingredient Flatbread _____ 84

3 Ingredient Keto Flatbread_____ 86

Tasty Keto Flatbread _____ 88

Almond Flour Tortillas _____ 90

Coconut Flour Tortillas_____ 92

Cheesy Flatbread _____ 94

Keto Tortillas _____ 96

Low Carb Tortilla_____ 98

Chapter 6: Other Keto Bread Recipes ___ 100

Low Carb Roll _____ 100

Almond Scones _____ 102

Ham & Cheese Pretzels _____ 105

Keto Breadsticks _____ 108

Keto Brioche Bread _____ 111

Low Carb Garlic Bread _____ 114

Sweet Challah Bread _____ 116

Cheesy Breadsticks _____ 118

Keto Scones _____ 121

Conclusion _____ 124

Introduction

Starting a new healthy lifestyle is usually exciting and most of us look forward to enjoying all the health benefits that come with a healthy lifestyle. However, like everything, within a few days, once the excitement wears off, it then dawns on you, the decision you have made and what it takes.

For example, the ketogenic diet requires that you limit your carbohydrate intake and carbohydrates like wheat, oats, rice, bread etc are off limits. Not eating such carbohydrates especially bread, which is something most people are used to can be okay for some days but after a few days, you are likely to crave for bread. How then do you ensure that you don't fall off the bandwagon? By finding suitable keto alternatives for foods that you like that, you cannot eat while on the ketogenic diet. One such food is bread.

To ensure that you stick to the keto diet and don't end up eating bread and you can stick with the keto lifestyle for the long haul, this book has over 60 different kinds of keto bread from loaves and bagels to muffins and cornbread. With so many recipes, you are definitely bound to find something you like.

Let us start with some keto buns and bagels:

Chapter 1: Keto Buns and Bagels

Keto Buns

Prep time: 5 minutes

Cook time: 40 minutes

Total time: 45 minutes

Yields: 4 servings

Ingredients

2 egg yolks

1 cup of water

½ tablespoon of apple cider vinegar

1 teaspoon of baking powder

4 egg whites

2 tablespoons of ground psyllium husks

¼ cup of coconut flour

Salt and pepper to taste

Optional:

1 teaspoon of dried thyme

Keto Bread

1 teaspoon of dried oregano

Directions

Preheat your oven to 350 degrees F.

Line a baking sheet with parchment paper.

Beat the egg whites using a whisk or a hand mixer until they foam stiff peaks then set aside.

In a separate bowl mix the remaining ingredients then gently fold in the egg whites.

Use the resulting dough to form 4 thick even sized rolls and place them on the prepared baking sheet. Ensure they are thick enough so that the buns do not flatten

Bake until cooked all the way through for around 40 minutes. Remove one bun from the oven and cut it open. If it is still moist, place them back in the oven (including the one you cut open) for a few more minutes.

Serve warm.

Nutritional info per serving: Calories 120, Protein 6g, Carbs 6g and Fats 3.1g

Almond Flour Buns

Prep time: 15 minutes

Cook time: 1 hour

Total time: 1 hour 15 minutes

Yields: 6 servings

Ingredients

1 teaspoon of sea salt

3 egg whites

1 cup of boiling water

2 teaspoons of apple cider vinegar

5 tablespoons of psyllium husk powder, ground

2 teaspoons of baking powder

1 ¼ cups of almond flour

Directions

Preheat your oven to 350 degrees F.

Combine all the dry ingredients in a bowl. Add in the cup of boiling water into the bowl then mix in the vinegar and the egg whites

Use a hand mixer to beat the ingredients together for around 30 seconds. Don't over mix. The resulting mix should have a Play Dough-like consistency.

Wet your hands then form the dough into 4-8 pieces. You can shape them into hot dog or hamburger buns according to your preference.

Grease your baking sheet with oil then place the formed dough on top. Place in the oven on the lower rack and bake for 50 to 60 minutes – depends on the size of your buns.

Tap the base of the bun to check if done. Remove from the oven if it produces a hollow sound. Serve with your favorite topping or butter

Store the leftovers in the freezer or fridge.

Nutritional info per serving: Calories 73, Protein 3.1g, Carbs 3g and Fat 2.8g

Tasty Keto Buns

Prep time: 10-15 minutes

Cook time: 45 minutes

Total time: 55 to 60 minutes

Yields: 10 buns

Ingredients

Dry ingredients

2 teaspoons cream of tartar or apple cider vinegar

1 teaspoon of baking soda

5 tablespoons of sesame seeds

1 teaspoon of sea salt or pink Himalayan salt

2 teaspoons of onion powder

2 teaspoons of garlic powder

½ packed cup of flax meal

½ cup of coconut flour

2/3 cup of psyllium husks or ½ cup of psyllium husk powder

1 ½ cups of almond flour (almond meal)

Keto Bread

Optional: 1-2 tablespoons of erythritol or swerve

Wet ingredients

2 cups of water (lukewarm or boiling depending on method)

2 large eggs

6 large egg whites

Directions

Preheat your oven to 350 degrees F.

Add the baking soda, cream of tartar, onion powder, garlic powder, salt, Psyllium powder, flax meal, coconut flour, almond flour (and optionally erythritol) to a mixing bowl.

*Don't use whole psyllium husks. If you cannot get psyllium husk powder, use a coffee grinder or a blender to process until fine

Add in the egg whites and eggs and use a hand mixer to process well until the dough is thick – we don't use whole eggs because too many yolks will prevent the buns from rising

Pour in the boiling water and process well until combined.

Use a spoon to make the buns then place them on a non-stick baking tray or a tray lined with parchment paper. Leave some space between them, as they will rise. You may also use small tart trays. Top with the sesame seeds (or any other seeds of your choosing) and press into the dough so that they don't fall out

Place the tray in the oven and cook for 45 to 50 minutes.

Remove from oven and allow the tray to cool down before placing the buns on a rack to cool to room temperature.

Store at room temperature if eating for the next couple of days or store in freezer for future use.

Top with burger meat, cream cheese or butter. Enjoy

Nutritional info per serving: Calories 208, Proteins 10.1g, Carbs 12.4g and Fats 15.2g

Fluffy Buns

Prep time: 5 minutes

Cook time: 25 minutes

Total time: 30 minutes

Yields: 4 servings

Ingredients

1 teaspoon of baking powder

1 tablespoon of psyllium husk powder

¼ cup of coconut flour

¼ cup of almond flour

¼ cup of boiling water

1 egg at room temp

3 egg whites at room temp

Optional: sesame seeds for sprinkling

Directions

Preheat your oven to 356 degrees F.

Keto Bread

Mix all the dry ingredients then place them in the food processor together with all the remaining ingredients or mix in an electric blender for about 20 seconds until smooth. Don't over mix.

Allow the dough to sit for a few minutes so that the flours absorb moisture.

Divide the dough into 4 equal portions then form the buns.

Prepare your baking sheet by lining it with parchment paper then place the buns on top. Sprinkle with sesame seeds or any other seeds of your choice.

On top of the buns, make a criss-cross cuts then bake until browned for around 25 minutes.

Nutritional info per serving: Calories 109, Protein 7.3g, Carbs 8.3g and Fat 5.5g

Cheesy Hamburger Buns

Prep time: 8 minutes

Cook time: 12 minutes

Total time: 20 minutes

Yields: 6 servings

Ingredients

4 tablespoons of melted grass fed butter

3 cups of almond flour

4 large eggs

4 oz cream cheese

2 cups of mozzarella cheese, shredded

Sesame seeds (each)

Directions

Preheat your oven to 400 degrees F.

Prepare a baking sheet by lining with parchment paper.

Melt together the cream cheese and mozzarella cheese. Add 3 of the eggs then stir to combine. Add in the almond flour and mix.

Keto Bread

Form 6 bun shaped balls from the dough then place onto the earlier prepared baking sheet.

Brush with the remaining egg and butter then sprinkle with sesame seeds.

Bake for 10 to 12 minutes until golden.

Nutritional info per serving: Calories 287, Protein 14.7g, Carbs 2.4g and Fats 25.8g

Ultimate Keto Buns

Prep time: 5 minutes

Cook time: 26 minutes

Total time: 31 minutes

Yields: 6 buns

Ingredients

1 teaspoon of onion flakes

1 tablespoon of black sesame seeds

1 tablespoon of white sesame seeds

1 tablespoon of rosemary

100g of blanched almond flour

½ teaspoon of Himalayan salt

4 eggs

4 tablespoons of melted lard

Directions

Preheat your oven to 43 degrees F.

Keto Bread

Add the eggs and melted lard to the stick blender beaker. Add in the remaining ingredients. Pulse until the batter is completely mixed for 5-10 times.

Divide the batter equally among 6 silicone jumbo muffin molds. Sprinkle the top of each bun with the extra sesame seeds. If you want the bun to be thicker, divide among 4 molds instead of 6.

Bake for 26 minutes then remove from oven and allow the buns to cool completely before cutting.

Nutritional info per serving: Calories 230, Protein 8.45g, Carbs 3.99g and Fat 20.82g

Keto Bagels

Prep time: 10 minutes

Cook time: 20 minutes

Total time: 30 minutes

Yields: 6 servings

Ingredients

1 teaspoon of baking powder

1 tablespoon of psyllium husk powder

4 tablespoons of cream cheese

1 large egg, beaten

1 cup of extra fine almond flour

1 ½ cups of shredded mozzarella

Sesame seeds/ poppy seeds (optional)

Directions

Preheat your oven to 360 degrees F / 180 C.

In a microwave, melt the cream cheese and mozzarella on high for 1 ½ minutes. You can also melt them in a non-stick pan

Keto Bread

In another separate bowl, mix the dry ingredients – baking powder, psyllium husk powder and almond flour.

Add the beaten egg and the dry ingredients mix to the melted cheeses then mix using a spatula. Use your hands to knead the mixture until you form smooth dough. Alternatively mix in a food processor or stand mixer.

Form a large ball then split into 6 segments. Make bagel shapes by forming the segments into logs then laying them down in a circle and pinching the ends together.

Prepare a baking sheet by lining with parchment paper then place the bagels on top. Sprinkle with sesame seeds or poppy seeds.

Bake until lightly browned on top for around 20 minutes.

Nutritional info per serving: Calories 231, Protein 12.8g, Carbs 6.6g and Fats 18.1g

Rosemary Bagels

Prep time: 10 minutes

Cook time: 45 minutes

Total time: 55 minutes

Yields: 6 servings

Ingredients

1 tablespoon of rosemary chopped

12 cup of warm water

3 egg whites

1 whole egg

3 tablespoons of psyllium husk powder

¼ teaspoon of salt

¾ teaspoon of xantham gum

¾ teaspoon of baking soda

1 ½ cups of almond flour

Avocado oil

Keto Bread

Directions

Preheat your oven to 250 degrees F.

In a bowl, mix the almond flour, salt, baking soda and xanthan gum.

Whisk together the warm water and eggs in a separate bowl then add in the psyllium husks and stir until there are no clumps.

Add the wet ingredients to the dry ingredients then use avocado oil to coat the bagel mold.

Press the dough into mold and sprinkle the rosemary on top.

Bake in the oven for 45 minutes then remove from the oven and let it sit for 15 minutes before slicing.

Nutritional info per serving: Calories 285, Proteins 13g, Carbs 12g and Fat 22.5g

Keto Bagel

Prep time: 2 minutes

Cook time: 15 minutes

Total time: 17 minutes

Yields: 6 servings

Ingredients

1 cup of any cheese that melts well, shredded (cheddar, mozzarella)

½ cup of grated parmesan

2 eggs

2 tablespoons of everything bagel seasoning

Directions

Preheat your oven to 375 degrees F.

In a bowl, combine the egg and the shredded cheese and mix until they are fully combined.

Portion the mixture into 6 parts then press onto a well greased donut pan. Sprinkle the everything bagel seasoning on the egg and cheese mixture.

Keto Bread

Bake until the cheese forms a slight brown crust and has fully melted (about 15 to 20 minutes).

Nutritional info per serving: Calories 218, Protein 14g, Carbs 5g and Fat 16g

Mozzarella Dough Bagels

Prep time: 10 minutes

Cook time: 15 minutes

Total time: 25 minutes

Yields: 6 servings

Ingredients

1 teaspoon of baking powder

1 egg, medium

2 tablespoons of full fat cream cheese

85g of almond flour/meal

170g of grated / pre shredded mozzarella cheese

Pinch of salt to taste

Directions

In a microwave safe bowl, mix the cream cheese, almond meal/flour and grated/ shredded cheese. Microwave for 1 minute on high.

Stir then place back in the oven and microwave for 30 more seconds on high.

Keto Bread

Add in the salt, baking powder, egg and any other flavorings then mix gently. Portion the dough into 6 equal parts and roll them into balls then into cylinder shapes. Fold the cylinder ends in a circle then squeeze the 2 ends to form a bagel shape.

Place onto a baking tray and sprinkle with sesame seeds.

Bake until golden brown for 15 minutes at 425 degrees F/ 220 C.

Nutritional info per serving: Calories 203, Protein 11g, Carbs 4g and Fat 16.8g

Chapter 2: Keto Muffins

Walnut Flax Muffins

Prep time: 10 minutes

Cook time: 20 minutes

Total time: 30 minutes

Yields: 12 muffins

Ingredients

½ teaspoon of baking soda

1 teaspoon of lemon juice

2 teaspoons of cinnamon

2 teaspoons of vanilla extract

¼ cup of coconut flour

½ cup of granulated sweetener

Pinch of sea salt

½ cup of avocado oil or any other oil

4 pastured eggs

Keto Bread

1 cup of ground golden flax seed or just buy already ground flax meal

Optional: 1 cup of chopped walnuts

Directions

Preheat your oven to 325 degrees F.

If using whole golden flax seed, place in a coffee grinder and grind then measure 1 cup.

In a mixing bowl, add in the ingredients as follows: ground flax seed/ flax meal, eggs, avocado oil, sweetener, coconut flour, vanilla, cinnamon, lemon juice, baking soda, sea salt and finally the chopped walnuts (if using). Mix everything until well combined. You may use an electric mixer but if you do, add the walnuts last.

Bake for 18 to 22 minutes.

Nutritional info per serving: Calories 219, Protein 6g, Carbs 6g and Fat 20g

Peanut Butter Muffins

Prep time: 20 minutes

Cook time: 25 minutes

Total time: 45 minutes

Yields: 6 servings

Ingredients

2 large eggs

1/3 cup of almond milk

1/3 cup of peanut butter

1 pinch of salt

½ cup of cacao nibs or sugar free chocolate chips

1 teaspoon of baking powder

12 cup of So Nourished erythritol

1 cup of almond flour

Directions

Preheat your oven to 350 degrees F.

Keto Bread

In a large mixing bowl, combine all dry ingredients apart from the cacao nibs (or sugar free chocolate chips) and stir.

Add in the almond milk and peanut butter then stir to combine. Add the eggs in one at a time stirring until fully combined before adding another. Fold in the cacao nibs.

Use cooking oil spray, spray a muffin tin then distribute the batter evenly to make six large muffins.

Bake for around 20 to 30 minutes then leave to completely cool.

Enjoy with a drizzle of sugar free maple syrup or butter

Nutritional info per serving: Calories 265, Protein 7.5g, Carbs 2g and Fat 20.5g

Chocolate Zucchini Muffins

Prep time: 10 minutes

Cook time: 30 minutes

Total time: 40 minutes

Yields: 9 muffins

Ingredients

1/3 cup of Lily's chocolate baking chips

¼ cup of heavy cream

1 medium zucchini grated

1 tablespoon of oil

2 teaspoons of vanilla extract

2/3 cup of swerve sweetener

3 large eggs

½ teaspoon of nutmeg

1 teaspoon of cinnamon

½ teaspoon of salt

2 tablespoons of cocoa powder

¾ teaspoon of baking soda

½ cup of coconut flour

Directions

Preheat your oven to 350 degrees F.

Line a muffin tin with cupcake liners then use cooking spray to spray the inside of the liners.

Combine the nutmeg, sweetener, cinnamon, salt, cocoa powder, baking soda and coconut flour in a bowl. Combine the zucchini, cream, oil, vanilla and eggs in a separate bowl.

Pour the wet ingredients over the dry ingredients and stir until combined then fold in the chocolate chips.

Scoop the batter into the lined muffin tins and bake until when you insert a toothpick it comes out clean (takes around 30 minutes).

Remove the pan from the oven and allow the muffins to cool in the pan

Nutritional info per serving: Calories 117, Protein 3.9g, Carbs 12.2g and Fat 7.7g

Keto Chocolate Muffins

Prep time: 10 minutes

Cook time: 20 minutes

Total time: 30 minutes

Yields: 12 muffins

Ingredients

½ cup of sugar free chocolate chips

3 ounces of unsalted butter, melted

2/3 cup of heavy cream

3 eggs

1 teaspoon of vanilla extract

1 ½ teaspoons of baking powder

½ cup of erythritol

½ cup of unsweetened cocoa powder

1 cup of almond flour

Directions

Preheat your oven to 350 degrees F.

Combine the baking powder, erythritol, cocoa powder and almond flour in a bowl.

Add in the heavy cream, eggs, vanilla and mix well. Add the melted butter and stir to combine. Add the chocolate chips then continue to stir.

Prepare a standard 12-count muffin tray by lining with cupcake papers then spoon the mixture into the tray.

Bake for around 20 minutes.

You can eat the muffins right away or allow them to cool in the muffin tin

Nutritional info per serving: Calories 301, Protein 7g, Carbs 9g and Fat 26g

Blackberry-Filled Keto Muffins

Prep time: 20 minutes

Cook time: 25 minutes

Total time: 45 minutes

Yields: 12 muffins

Ingredients

For the blackberry filling:

1 cup of frozen or fresh blackberries

1 tablespoon of lemon juice

2 tablespoons of water

¼ teaspoon of xanthan gum

3 tablespoons of granulated Stevia erythritol

For the muffin batter:

½ teaspoon of lemon extract

1 teaspoon of vanilla extract

¼ cup of coconut oil, ghee or butter melted

¼ cup of unsweetened almond milk

Keto Bread

4 large eggs

1 teaspoon of grain free baking powder

½ teaspoon of salt

1 teaspoon of fresh lemon zest

¾ cup of erythritol blend / granulated Stevia

2 ½ cups of superfine almond flour

Directions

For the blackberry filling:

Whisk together the xanthan gum and granulated sweetener in a 1 ½-quart saucepan. Add the lemon juice and water a tablespoon at a time stirring between additions.

Stir in the blackberries then heat over medium low heat. Bring to a simmer stirring frequently then turn the heat to low. Simmer for about 10 minutes until the blackberries break up and form a thick jam like syrup then remove from heat. Allow the mixture to cool

For the muffin batter:

Preheat your oven to 350 degrees F.

Line a muffin pan with muffin paper and set aside.

Whisk together the baking powder, sea salt, lemon zest, granulated sweetener and almond flour in a medium bowl.

Whisk together the lemon extract, vanilla extract, almond milk and eggs in a small bowl then stream in the butter while whisking.

Pour the wet ingredients over the dry ingredients slowly while stirring then spoon the batter onto the earlier prepared muffin cups to be around 1/3 full.

Use a spoon or clean fingers to form a depression in the batter cups then in each depression, pour a spoonful of the cooled blackberry jam. Use the remaining batter to cover the blackberry jam so that each cup is 2/3 full

Bake until the tops spring back when lightly touched for around 25 to 30 minutes.

Store the leftovers in an airtight container in the fridge or refrigerator.

Nutritional info per serving: Calories 199, Protein 7g, Carbs 4g and Fat 17g

Coffee Cake Muffins

Prep time: 15 minutes

Cook time: 35 minutes

Total time: 55 minutes

Yields: 12 servings

Ingredients

Crumb topping:

¼ cup of butter, melted

¾ teaspoon of cinnamon

2 tablespoons of coconut flour

3 tablespoons of swerve brown

½ cup of almond flour

Muffins:

½ teaspoon of vanilla extract

½ cup of almond milk, unsweetened

4 large eggs

½ cup of butter, melted

¼ teaspoon of salt

½ teaspoon of cinnamon

1 tablespoon of baking powder

3 tablespoons of coconut flour

¼ cup of whey protein powder, unflavored

1/3 cup of swerve sweetener

2 cups of almond flour

Drizzle:

½ teaspoon of vanilla extract

2 tablespoons of water

¼ cup of powdered swerve sweetener

Directions

Topping:

Whisk together the cinnamon, coconut flour, swerve and almond flour together in a medium bowl. Pour in the melted butter and stir well to combine. Set aside.

Muffins:

Preheat your oven to 325 degrees F.

Keto Bread

Prepare a standard muffin tin by lining with silicone liners or parchment paper then set aside.

Whisk together the almond flour, salt, cinnamon, coconut flour, protein powder and sweetener in a large bowl. Stir in the vanilla, almond milk, eggs and butter until well combined.

Divide the batter equally among the earlier prepared muffin cups then top with the crumb topping.

Bake until when a toothpick inserted in comes out clean or for around 25 to 35 minutes

Leave in the pan to cool completely.

Drizzle:

Whisk together the vanilla, water and sweetener. If the resulting mixture is too thick, add more water. Drizzle over the cooled muffins lightly

Nutritional info per serving: Calories 285, Protein 9.1g, Carbs 7.6g and Fat 24.4g

Keto Blueberry Muffins

Prep time: 10 minutes

Cook time: 20 minutes

Total time: 30 minutes

Yields: 12 muffins

Ingredients

¾ cup of blueberries

½ teaspoon of vanilla extract

3 large eggs

1/3 cup of unsweetened almond milk

1/3 cup of coconut oil or butter (measured in solid form then melted)

¼ teaspoon of sea salt (optional – recommended)

1 ½ teaspoons of gluten free baking powder

½ cup of erythritol (or any other granulated sweetener)

2 ½ cups of blanched almond flour

Keto Bread

Directions

Preheat your oven to 350 degrees F.

Prepare your muffin pan by lining with 12 parchment paper or silicone muffin liners.

Stir together the sea salt, baking powder, erythritol and almond flour in a large bowl. Mix in the vanilla extract, eggs, almond milk and melted coconut oil then fold in the blueberries.

Divide the batter equally among the lined muffin cups and bake for about 20 to 25 minutes or until when you insert a toothpick, it comes out clean and the top is brown.

Nutritional info per serving: Calories 217, Protein 7g, Carbs 6g and Fat 19g

Chapter 3: Keto Loaves

Fluffy Keto Bread Loaf

Prep time: 15 minutes

Cook time: 45 minutes

Total time: 1 hour

Yields: 12 servings

Ingredients

½ teaspoon of sea salt

½ teaspoon of xanthan gum

1 teaspoon of baking powder

2 cups of blanched almond flour

2 tablespoons of olive oil

12 cup of butter, melted and cooled

7 eggs at room temp

Cooking spray

Directions

Preheat your oven to 350 degrees F.

Keto Bread

Prepare your silicone loaf pan by greasing with cooking spray.

In a bowl, whisk all the eggs for about 3 minutes until creamy and smooth. Add in the olive oil and melted butter and mix until well combined.

In a separate bowl, combine the almond flour, salt, xanthan gum and baking powder. Mix well then gradually add it to the egg mixture. Mix well until you form a thick batter.

Pour the batter onto the greased pan then use a spatula to smooth the top

Bake for about 45 minutes until a toothpick comes out clean when inserted into the centre

Nutritional info per serving: Calories 247, Proteins 7.7g, Carbs 4.9g and Fats 22.8g

Dairy Free Keto Loaf

Prep time: 5 minutes

Cook time: 30 minutes

Total time: 35 minutes

Yields: 12 servings

Ingredients

½ teaspoon of salt

2 teaspoons of baking soda

¼ cup of melted butter or coconut oil

¼ cup of water or almond milk

½ cup of chia seeds (preferably white)

1 cup of almond flour

4 eggs

Directions

Preheat your oven to 350 degrees F.

Grease an 8 x 4 inch loaf pan and set aside. (*note: don't use a larger loaf pan since the bread is going to be very flat. If you want your bread to rise more, bake in 2 mini pans)

Keto Bread

In a bowl combine all ingredients and stir until the batter is not lumpy and is well mixed

Pour the batter onto the earlier prepared loaf pan and bake for 30 minutes. Leave the bread in the pan to rest for 10 minutes before removing and placing on a rack if you want to cool it completely. If not, just enjoy it right away with some butter

Nutritional info per serving: Calories 148, Protein 5g, Carbs 5g and Fat 12g

Simple Almond Flour Bread

Prep time: 10 minutes

Cook time: 45 minutes

Total time: 55 minutes

Yields: 12 slices

Ingredients

2 cups of almond flour

7 eggs

2 tablespoons of coconut oil

½ cup of butter

Directions

Preheat your oven to 350 degrees F.

Prepare a loaf pan by lining it with parchment paper.

In a bowl, mix the eggs for up to 2 minutes on high. Add in the melted butter, almond flour and melted coconut oil then continue to mix.

Pour the mixture onto the earlier prepared loaf pan.

Bake until a toothpick comes out clean when you insert in the loaf or for around 45-50 minutes.

Nutritional info per serving: Calories 178, Protein 6.4g, Carbs 3.9g and Fats 15g

Keto Bread

Prep time: 15 minutes

Cook time: 40 minutes

Total time: 55 minutes

Yields: 16 slices

Ingredients

½ teaspoon of salt

½ teaspoon of Xanthan gum

200g of almond flour

1 teaspoon of baking powder

7 large eggs

30g of coconut oil

1g of butter, melted

Directions

Preheat your oven to 355 degrees F (180c).

Beat the eggs in a bowl for 1 to 2 minutes on high. Add in the melted butter and coconut oil and continue beating. Add the rest of the ingredients; the resulting batter is going to be quite thick.

Prepare your loaf pan by lining with baking paper then scrape the mix into the pan.

Bake until a skewer comes out of the loaf clean or for 45 minutes.

Slice into 16 thin slices then store in the fridge in an airtight container for up to a week or in the freezer for up to a month.

Nutritional info per serving: Calories 165, Protein 6g, Carbs 3g and Fat 15g

Best Keto Bread

Prep time: 10 minutes

Cook time: 30 minutes

Total time: 40 minutes

Yields: 20 slices

Ingredients

1 pinch of pink salt

3 teaspoons of baking powder

¼ cup of butter, melted

6 large eggs, separated

1 ½ cup of almond flour

Optional:

6 drops of liquid Stevia

¼ teaspoon cream of tartar

Directions

Preheat your oven to 375 degrees F.

Keto Bread

Separate the egg yolks and egg whites. To the egg whites, add the cream of tartar and beat until you achieve soft peaks.

Combine the almond flour, salt, baking powder, melted butter, 1/3 of the beaten egg whites and the egg yolks in a food processor (adding the liquid Stevia helps in reducing the mild taste of egg). Mix until combined; you will have a lumpy thick dough

Add in the remaining 2/3 of your whites and process gently until fully incorporated. Ensure that you don't over mix as this resulting mixture is what gives the bread its volume.

Transfer the mixture to a buttered 8x4-inch loaf pan and bake for around 30 minutes.

Nutritional info per serving: Calories 90, Protein 3g, Carbs 2g and Fats 7g

Sesame Seed Keto Bread

Prep time: 10 minutes

Cook time: 1 hour 5 minutes

Total time: 1 hour 15 minutes

Yields: 10 servings

Ingredients

3 egg whites

1 cup of boiling water

2 teaspoons of apple cider vinegar

1 teaspoon of salt

2 teaspoons of baking powder

5 tablespoons of psyllium husk powder

1 ¼ cups (143g) of almond flour

2 tablespoons of sesame seeds

Directions

Preheat your oven to 350 degrees F.

Keto Bread

Prepare a 9x5 inch loaf tin by lining it with parchment paper then butter and set aside.

Combine the salt, psyllium husk powder, baking powder and almond flour in a large bowl. Add the apple cider vinegar and egg whites to the dry ingredients and mix using an electric mixer on medium speed until a paste-like dough forms

Add in the boiling water while mixing on low speed. Increase speed to high and mix until a play-dough like mixture forms. Do not over mix.

Place the dough onto the earlier prepared baking tin then smooth the top. Sprinkle with the sesame seeds .

Bake until the top rises and puffs up like a traditional sandwich loaf.

Once done, remove the bread from the oven and leave it to slightly cool before moving it to a cooling rack

Slice and enjoy once cool.

Store the leftovers covered at room temperature for up to 2 days.

Nutritional info per serving: Calories 53, Protein 2g, Carbs 4g and Fat 3g

Low Carb Bread

Prep time: 15 minutes

Cook time: 1 hour 30 minutes

Total time: 1 hour 45 minutes

Yields: 14 servings

Ingredients

1 teaspoon of sesame seeds

¾ cup of boiling water

6 tablespoons of butter ghee, grass-fed clarified – melted then cooled slightly

5 drops of liquid Stevia

2 tablespoons of apple cider vinegar

1 cup of egg whites at room temp

3 tablespoons of boiling water

1 tablespoon of grass-fed beef gelatin

2 teaspoons of coconut sugar

2 tablespoons of warm water

Keto Bread

2 teaspoons of instant yeast

2 teaspoons of baking powder

1 teaspoon of salt

2 tablespoons of psyllium husk powder

¾ cup of coconut flour

2 cups of almond flour

Avocado oil spray for the pan

Directions

Preheat your oven to 350 degrees F.

Use parchment paper to line a 9 by 5 inch loaf pan then spray the inside lightly with avocado oil.

In a large bowl, whisk together the baking powder, salt, psyllium husk powder, coconut flour and almond flour.

In a small bowl, stir together the coconut sugar, 2 tablespoons of warm water and yeast then let it sit until foamy for about 10 minutes.

In another small bowl whisk together 3 tablespoons of boiling water and gelatin until fully dissolved.

Keto Bread

In a medium bowl, stir together the melted ghee, Stevia, vinegar, egg whites, dissolved beef gelatin and dissolved yeast.

Pour the egg mixture into the dry ingredients mixture then stir in ¾ cup of boiling water. Pour the resulting mixture onto the earlier prepared pan and smooth the top. Let it sit for 3 minutes then top with sesame seeds.

Bake for 75 minutes to 90 minutes until a toothpick comes out clean when inserted. You will know the loaf is done if when you tap it at the bottom, it produces a hollow sound.

Switch off the oven and leave the oven door ajar for the bread to cool in the warm oven for around 30 minutes.

Transfer the bread to a wire rack until done cooling before slicing

Nutritional info per serving: Calories 198, Protein 7g, Carbs 9g and Fat 15g

Chapter 4: Keto "Cornbread" Recipes

Sweet Keto Cornbread

Prep time: 10 minutes

Cook time: 45 minutes

Total time: 55 minutes

Yields: 12 servings

Ingredients

3 eggs

1 teaspoon of xanthan gum

4 tablespoons of baking powder

2 tablespoons erythritol sweetener

1/3 cup of coconut flour

¾ cup of super fine almond flour

2 tablespoons of butter

4 oz of cream cheese

2 cups of part-skim mozzarella cheese, shredded

15-20 drops of cornbread flavoring oil

Keto Bread

Directions

Preheat your oven to 350 degrees F.

Prepare an 8×8 inch baking dish by greasing with butter.

Combine the butter, cream cheese and mozzarella cheese in a large microwave safe bowl. Microwave in 30 second increments stirring in between each until the mixture is smooth and melted; this takes around 2-3 minutes

Remove from the microwave then add in the xanthan gum, baking powder, sweetener, coconut flour and almond flour. Stir to combine and return to the microwave once the cheeses begin to harden

Add the cornbread flavoring and eggs and mix to combine. Transfer onto the earlier prepared baking dish once all ingredients are mixed together well and cover with aluminum foil.

Bake for 30 minutes then uncover and bake for 10-15 more minutes or until the bread springs back when pushed lightly and the top is golden brown.

Allow the bread to slightly cool before you slice it up and serve.

Keto Bread

Nutritional info per serving: Calories 180, Protein 8g, Carbs 5g and Fat 13g

Low Carb Cornbread Muffins

Prep time: 15 minutes

Cook time: 25 minutes

Total time: 40 minutes

Yields: 12 servings

Ingredients

1/8 teaspoon of salt

1 ½ teaspoons of baking powder

3 tablespoons of swerve confectioners

¼ cup of almond meal

1 cup of coconut flour

3 oz of cream cheese, softened

5 tablespoons of salted butter, melted

½ cup of unsweetened coconut milk (from a carton)

½ cup of heavy whipping cream

3 eggs, beaten slightly

Keto Bread

Directions

Preheat your oven to 350 degrees F.

If using a silicone muffin pan like this recipe does, you don't need to grease it. However, if not using silicone, use liners or grease the pan lightly for easy removal.

In a large bowl, combine the cream cheese, melted butter (slightly cooled), coconut milk, whipping cream and the eggs. Mix everything using a hand mixer until the cream cheese is incorporated well (it is okay to have a few small flecks), and set aside.

Combine the baking powder, swerve confectioners, salt, almond meal and coconut flour in a medium sized bowl, and mix thoroughly

Add the dry ingredients to the wet ingredients then use a hand mixer to mix thoroughly.

Distribute the batter evenly among the holes pressing it down a bit with the back of a spoon.

Bake for 20-25 minutes until a toothpick comes out clean when inserted and the edges start to brown.

Be careful not to over-bake. The centre should come out slightly soft but not uncooked

Cool and enjoy.

Nutritional info per serving: Calories 169, Protein 4g, Carbs 7.8g and Fat 14g

Keto "Cornbread"

Prep time: 5 minutes

Cook time: 30 minutes

Total time: 35 minutes

Yields: 16 servings

Ingredients

¼ cup of butter, melted

½ cup of heavy cream

3 large eggs

½ teaspoon of baking soda

1 teaspoon of salt

¼ cup of coconut flour

½ cup of almond flour

Optional fillings:

½ cup of shredded cheddar cheese

4 slices of bacon, cooked and crumbled

2 jalapenos, sliced thinly

Directions

Preheat your oven to 325 degrees F.

Mix all the ingredients apart from the jalapenos in a medium sized bowl (simply omit the fillings if you don't want to use them).

Pour the batter into a well-greased 10.5" cast iron skillet then top with the jalapenos. Bake for around 25 to 30 minutes then allow the bread to cool for 5 minutes before cutting.

You can store the bread for up to 3 days at room temperature.

Nutritional info per serving: Calories 120, Protein 4.1g, Carbs 1.5g and Fats 10.8g

Low Carb Cornbread

Prep time: 10 minutes

Cook time: 20 minutes

Total time: 30 minutes

Yields: 8 slices of bread

Ingredients

¼ teaspoon of baking soda

12 teaspoon of salt

2 tablespoons of monkfruit sweetener

½ cup of coconut flour

3 large eggs

1/3 cup of heavy cream

6 tablespoons of butter, melted

Directions

Preheat your oven to 350 degrees F.

Spray an 8 by 8 baking dish or a 10-inch iron cast skillet with non-stick cooking spray.

Keto Bread

In a mixing bowl whisk together the eggs, cream and melted butter until fully combined.

Add in the baking soda, salt, sweetener and coconut flour and stir to combine.

Pour the mixture onto the earlier prepared dish and bake until a toothpick comes out clean and the edges are golden (around 15 to 20 minutes).

Nutritional info per serving: Calories 167, Protein 4g, Carbs 4g and Fat 15g

Almond Flour "Cornbread"

Prep time: 15 minutes

Cook time: 25 minutes

Total time: 40 minutes

Yields: 9 slices

Ingredients

1 teaspoon of vanilla extract

1 teaspoon of baking powder

5 tablespoons of salted butter, melted – plus more for greasing the pan

4 large eggs

1/3 cup of confectioners Swerve

1 ½ cups of blanched almond flour

Optional for serving:

Sugar-free syrup

Slices of butter

Keto Bread

Directions

Preheat your oven to 350 degrees F.

Line an 8 by 8 inch baking dish with parchment paper and grease its sides.

Whisk together the baking powder, sweetener and almond flour in a mixing bowl.

Add the vanilla, melted butter and eggs in a separate mixing bowl and use a stand mixer or an electric mixer to beat the ingredients on low speed for about 30 seconds until well mixed.

Pour the flour mixture into the egg mixture and beat for about 30 seconds on low speed until smooth and incorporated. The resulting batter should be thick.

Pour the batter onto the earlier prepared pan then use a spatula to smooth the surface and to spread the batter to the corners and edges.

Bake for about 25 minutes until a toothpick comes out clean when inserted.

Allow the cornbread to cool for 5 minutes in the pan then release it by sliding a knife around the edges.

Keto Bread

Cut into 9 squares then serve warm with slices of butter or sugar free maple syrup

Nutritional info per serving: Calories 200, Protein 7g, Carbs 3.5g and Fat 18g

Tasty Keto Cornbread

Prep time: 10 minutes

Cook time: 13 minutes

Total time: 23 minutes

Yields: 8 servings

Ingredients

3 eggs

1/3 teaspoon of salt

1 teaspoon of baking powder

4 tablespoons of butter, melted

¾ cup of cheddar cheese, shredded

1 1/4 cups of almond flour

Directions

Preheat your oven to 400 degrees F.

If cooking with a cast iron skillet, place in the oven while it heats up and remove once the oven reaches 400 degrees F.

In a large bowl, combine all dry ingredients.

Keto Bread

Add in the wet ingredients and whisk until combined. Don't worry if the batter is lumpy.

Pour the batter onto the prepared muffin tins or the hot iron skillet.

Bake until golden brown for 15 to 20 minutes.

Store for up to a week in an airtight container

Nutritional info per serving: Calories 150, Protein 5.8g, Carbs 2.4g and Fat 13.4g

Simple Keto Cornbread

Prep time: 10 minutes

Cook time: 35 minutes

Total time: 45 minutes

Yields: 10 servings

Ingredients

1 teaspoon of sea salt

3 tablespoons of confectioners swerve

1/2 cup of melted butter plus 1 tablespoon for greasing the skillet

1 cup of sour cream

4 tablespoons of heavy whipping cream

4 eggs, beaten

2 teaspoons of baking powder

2 cups of almond meal

Directions

Preheat your oven to 375 degrees F.

Keto Bread

Combine the baking powder, salt and almond meal in a medium bowl then set aside.

Combine the eggs, sour cream and heavy cream in a medium bowl until fully combined.

Pour the wet ingredient into the dry ingredients and stir gently until fully incorporated then add in the melted butter and stir until mixed.

Into a preheated cast iron, add a teaspoon of butter then add in the batter. Bake for 30-35 minutes and serve warm or hot at room temperature.

Nutritional info per serving: Calorie 367, Protein 7.3g, Carbs 5.4 and Fat 36.6g

Chapter 5: Keto Flatbread and Tortilla Recipes

Keto Flatbread

Prep time: 2 minutes

Cook time: 20 minutes

Total time: 22 minutes

Yields: 6 servings

Ingredients

1/8 teaspoon of garlic powder

¼ cup spinach, cooked and drained

2 tablespoons of almond flour

1 egg

1 tablespoon of cream cheese

¾ cup of shredded mozzarella cheese

Salt to taste

Directions

Preheat your oven to 350 degrees F.

Keto Bread

Melt the cream cheese and mozzarella cheese in a microwave-safe bowl, in the microwave in 30-second increments mixing in between intervals to combine.

Mix in the spinach, almond flour and the egg, once the cheeses have melted completely and combined.

Prepare your baking sheet by lining with parchment paper then flatten the mixture out on top. Sprinkle the top with salt and garlic powder.

Bake the flatbread for 15 minutes then flip it over and cook the other side for 5 more minutes until crisp

Nutritional info per serving: Calories 65, Protein 5g, Carbs 1g and Fat 5g

Indian Flatbread

Prep time: 5 minutes

Cook time: 12 minutes

Total time: 17 minutes

Yields: 2 servings

Ingredients

½ cup of boiling water

1 teaspoon of beef gelatin dissolved in a tablespoon of boiling water

1 ½ tablespoons of coconut oil or ghee

1/8 teaspoon of salt

1/8 teaspoon of baking powder

½ tablespoon of psyllium husk powder

3 tablespoons of coconut flour

Directions

In a medium bowl, whisk together the baking powder, salt, psyllium husk powder and coconut flour.

Beat in the dissolved gelatin, boiling water and ghee until it forms dough

Portion the dough into 2 balls then place each between 2 pieces of plastic wrap or parchment paper and flatten into a 5 inch circle.

Preheat your non-stick skillet over medium high heat then add in some ghee. Add one of the dough circles into the skillet once the ghee is melted then reduce the heat to medium. Cook for about 12 minutes until both sides are golden, flipping as necessary

To prevent burning, you can turn the heat down a bit. You can cook the second dough the same way in a different skillet or wait until the first flatbread is ready then use that same skillet

Nutritional info per serving: Calories 190, Protein 3g, Carbs 8g and Fat 16g

Low-Carb Flatbread

Prep time: 5 minutes

Cook time: 5 minutes

Total time: 10 minutes

Yields: 6 servings

Ingredients

6 teaspoons of butter

1 pinch of sea salt

½ cup of arrowroot flour/powder

½ cup plus a heaping tablespoon of almond flour or coconut flour

1 cup of full fat coconut milk

Garnish (optional)

Directions

Whisk together all ingredients in a large bowl. It should have the consistency of pancake, loose and thick. If it's too loose/thin add single tablespoons of arrowroot flour and almond flour to thicken it. If it is too thick, add a single tablespoon of the coconut milk to thin out.

Keto Bread

Preheat a nonstick skillet on medium high heat then spray with a bit of olive oil.

Add a cup of the batter to the middle of the skillet. Cook the flatbread until firm and the edges are slightly brown but not crispy; this should take about 3 minutes.

Use a spatula to flip the flatbread and bake the other side for 2 to 3 more minutes until both sides are golden brown. Repeat this for the remaining flatbread dough.

Once done, cool the flatbread on a cooling rack. While still hot, brush the bread with the buttery spread. Enjoy with your desired topping.

Store any leftovers in the fridge for around 6 to 7 days

Nutritional info per serving: Calories 167, Proteins 2g, Carbs 13g and Fats 13g

5-ingredient Flatbread

Prep time: 5 minutes

Cook time: 20 minutes

Total time: 25 minutes

Yields: 8 servings

Ingredients

1 teaspoon of basil

1 tablespoon of garlic powder

2 tablespoons of almond flour

1 egg

1 tablespoon of cream cheese

¾ cup of mozzarella cheese

Directions

Preheat your oven to 350 degrees F.

Melt the cream cheese and mozzarella, and mix in the almond flour and the egg.

Prepare your baking sheet by lining with parchment paper then flatten the mixture on top.

Keto Bread

Sprinkle with the garlic powder and bake for 20 minutes.

Nutritional info per serving: Calories 56, Protein 3.6g, Carbs 0.8g and Fat 4.5g

3 Ingredient Keto Flatbread

Prep time: 2 minutes

Cook time: 24 minutes

Total time: 26 minutes

Yields: 8 servings

Ingredients

½ teaspoon of baking powder

8 egg whites

½ cup of almond flour

Optional:

Spices and herbs – thyme, red pepper flakes, basil, rosemary, garlic powder and salt (a teaspoon of each)

Coconut oil or Cooking spray

Directions

Whisk the egg whites lightly in a medium bowl then add the spices, salt, baking powder and almond flour. Whisk until there are no lumps.

Keto Bread

Spray your pan with coconut oil then add about ½ cup of the batter and cover with a lid.

Cook until the bread becomes bubbly and airy for about 2 minutes then flip the bread. Cook for another minute. Repeat this with the remaining batter.

Nutritional info per serving: Calories 57, Proteins 5g, Carbs 1.7g and Fat 3.6g

Tasty Keto Flatbread

Prep time: 15 minutes

Cook time: 25 minutes

Total time: 40 minutes

Yields: 6 servings

Ingredients

½ tablespoon of dried rosemary

½ tablespoon of black pepper corns

¼ teaspoon of granulated garlic

½ teaspoon of sea salt

1/3 cup of grated mozzarella cheese or parmesan cheese

1 cup of boiling water

¼ cup of olive oil

1 tablespoon of ground psyllium husk powder

½ cup of coconut flour

Keto Bread

Directions

In a mixing bowl, whisk together the dry ingredients then add the cheese and olive oil.

Add the hot water last while stirring and continue to stir until the coconut flour and psyllium fiber absorb all the water.

Line your baking sheet with parchment paper then press the dough onto the lined sheet until it is even and thin – keep the thickness less than 1/8 inch thick.

Bake for 20 to 25 minutes at 350 degrees F – the time depends on the thickness of your dough.

Transfer to a cooling rack once browned then remove the parchment paper and leave the flatbread to cool.

Cut the flatbread into squares using a pizza cutter for sandwiches.

If there are any leftovers store them in the refrigerator.

Nutritional info per serving: Calories 149, Protein 5g, Carbs 2g and Fat 12g

Almond Flour Tortillas

Prep time: 15 minutes

Cook time: 5 minutes

Total time: 20 minutes

Yields: 8 servings

Ingredients

120 ml boiling water

4 egg whites

1.5 teaspoons of salt

1 teaspoon of baking powder

6 tablespoons of psyllium husk powder

150g of blanched almond flour

1-2 tablespoons of oil for frying

Directions

In a large bowl, mix all the dry ingredients.

Add in the egg whites and mix well. Add in the boiling water, a little at a time and mix using a silicone spatula – as you mix, the psyllium absorbs the water.

Keto Bread

Let the dough sit for 5 minutes once you are done mixing then divide the dough into 8 balls.

Place the balls one at a time onto a piece of parchment paper then cover with another parchment paper.

Place your heaviest frying pan or skillet over the dough and press. Once pressed you may even twist the pan right to left to expand the dough. The tortillas will look thin however, they will thicken a bit once you cook them. Repeat this with the remaining dough.

Heat the cooking oil in a skillet or frying pan and place the tortillas in one at a time. Cook on medium heat for 20 to 40 seconds on each side until the crusts are golden brown.

Transfer to a plate once cooked to let them cool.

Nutritional info per serving: Calories 138, Protein 5.82g, Carbs 10.14g and Fat 9.4g

Coconut Flour Tortillas

Prep time: 5 minutes

Cook time: 10 minutes

Total time: 15 minutes

Yields: 4 servings

Ingredients

1 tablespoon of ghee or oil for frying

1 cup of water

½ teaspoon of baking powder

8g psyllium husk

50g coconut flour

Salt to taste

Directions

In a microwave safe bowl, heat 1 cup of water in the microwave for 30 seconds.

Mix all dry ingredients in a bowl and add the warm water. Knead to form dough then let it stand for 10 minutes then portion the dough into 4 parts.

Place one part of the dough between 2 pieces of parchment paper and roll it out.

Add a bit of ghee or butter to a pan then place the flat dough in the pan.

Allow the bottom side to cook completely before flipping to the other side. Ensure you cook both sides until golden brown.

Serve.

Nutritional info per serving: Calories 58, Protein 2g, Carbs 12g and Fat 2g

Cheesy Flatbread

Prep time: 5 minutes

Cook time: 15 minutes

Total time: 20 minutes

Yields: 6 servings

Ingredients

½ cup of grated cheddar cheese

1 egg

2 tablespoons of cream cheese, cubed

2 teaspoons of spicy seasoning

1 pinch of salt

6 tablespoons of almond flour

¾ cup of grated mozzarella

½ tablespoon of olive oil

Directions

Preheat your oven to 400 degrees F.

Keto Bread

Prepare your baking sheet by lining with parchment paper then brush with oil evenly. Set aside.

Mix the seasoning, sea salt, almond flour and mozzarella in a medium bowl then add in the cubed cream cheese on top.

Microwave for 45 seconds on high and stir then microwave for 20 more seconds and stir again. Add the egg and mix until fully combined

Place the dough onto the earlier prepared baking sheet and form a rectangle with the dough using your hands. Sprinkle with the cheddar evenly.

Bake until the cheese has melted and the bread has began to brown; this takes about 15 to 18 minutes

Slice and enjoy.

Nutritional info per serving: Calories 161, Protein 8.1g, Carbs 2.1g and Fat 13.8g

Keto Tortillas

Prep time: 20 minutes

Cook time: 10 minutes

Total time: 30 minutes

Yields: 8 servings

Ingredients

1 tablespoon of water

1 egg, beaten lightly

3 teaspoons of lime juice

½ teaspoon of kosher salt

1 teaspoon of baking powder

2 teaspoons of xanthan gum

¼ cup of coconut flour

1 cup of almond flour

Directions

In the bowl of a food processor, mix the baking powder, salt, xanthan gum, coconut flour and almond flour and pulse until combined for 5 seconds.

Keto Bread

Pour the lime into the flour mixture slowly with the food processor running then add the egg and water.

When the dough comes together to form a ball, transfer to a plastic wrap and tightly wrap it.

Knead the dough in your hands for 1-2 minutes then allow it to rest in the refrigerator for 10 minutes.

Divide the dough into 8 small balls of about 1 ½" diameter each. Place one ball between 2 wax papers or parchment paper and roll it to a thickness of about 1/8".

Over medium high heat, heat a large cast iron skillet then add the tortilla once hot and cook for about 20 seconds per side until slightly charred.

Repeat this with the remaining dough and serve immediately once done cooking.

Nutritional info per serving: Calories 27, Protein 1.2g, Carbs 0.9g and Fat 2.1gg

Low Carb Tortilla

Prep time: 10 minutes

Cook time: 12 minutes

Total time: 22 minutes

Yields: 6 servings

Ingredients

¼ teaspoon of onion powder

¼ teaspoon of garlic powder

½ teaspoon of salt

2 large eggs

6 ounces of shredded cheddar cheese

16 ounces of raw cauliflower (about half of a large head)

Directions

Preheat your oven to 400 degrees F.

Prepare several baking sheets by lining with parchment paper then set aside.

Chop the cauliflower lightly then place in the food processor. Pulse until the cauliflower is ground into crumbs then add in the remaining ingredients. Pulse until all ingredients combine.

Portion the mixture onto the earlier prepared baking sheets using a 3-tablespoon cookie scoop. Leave plenty of room to roll out the dough.

Use a piece of wax paper to cover the mounds then roll them into circles of about 4- 4 ½ inches and then remove the wax paper.

Bake until the tortillas are golden for 12 minutes then let them sit in the baking sheet for 3 to 5 minutes to cool.

Peel off the parchment paper. Enjoy

Nutritional info per serving: Calories 160, Protein 10g, Carbs 4g and Fat 11g

Chapter 6: Other Keto Bread Recipes

Low Carb Roll

Prep time: 5 minutes

Cook time: 13 minutes

Total time: 18 minutes

Yields: 8 servings

Ingredients

1 ¼ cups of almond flour

1 teaspoon of baking soda

2 tablespoons of plain whey protein isolate

1 large egg

2 ounces of cream cheese, cubed

1 ½ cups of shredded part skim mozzarella cheese

Directions

In a microwave safe bowl, melt the cream cheese and mozzarella together in the microwave for 1 minute. Stir then microwave for 30-45 more seconds. Transfer this to a food processor and process until mixed thoroughly.

Keto Bread

Add the eggs and mix again. Into the egg cheese mixture, add the dry ingredients and process for 10 to 15 seconds until thoroughly combined – should be very sticky.

Spray cooking oil on a piece of cling film then pour the bread dough at the center. Shape the dough gently into a rectangle or disk then freeze to cool as you prepare the oven. *Your dough does not need to go to the freezer if it is not very sticky.

Preheat your oven to 400 degrees F then place the rack in the middle of the oven. Prepare a cookie sheet by lining with silpat or a piece of parchment.

Remove the dough from the fridge and cut into 8 pieces. Oil your hands lightly then roll a portion of dough gently into a ball. Place the ball onto the prepared cookie sheet and flatten at the bottom. Repeat this with the remaining dough then sprinkle with dehydrated onion, poppy seeds or sesame seeds pressing gently into the dough.

Bake until the dough browns for approximately 13 to 15 minutes. It may also split.

Store the extra rolls in the fridge and warm before serving.

Nutritional info per serving: Calories 165, Protein 10g, Carbs 3g and Fat 13g

Almond Scones

Prep time: 15 minutes

Cook time: 25 minutes

Total time: 40 minutes

Yields: 8 servings

Ingredients

¼ cup of slivered almonds

1 teaspoon of orange extract

¼ cup of melted butter

¼ cup of heavy whipping cream

1 large egg

¼ teaspoon of sea salt

1 teaspoon of baking powder

¼ cup of swerve

¼ cup of coconut flour

1 cup of almond flour

For the glaze:

Keto Bread

3 tablespoons of powdered swerve

1 tablespoon of butter

1 tablespoon of cream cheese

Directions

Preheat your oven to 350 degrees F.

Prepare a cookie sheet by lining with parchment paper then set aside.

Whisk together the swerve, baking powder, coconut flour and almond flour in a large bowl then make a well in the mixture.

Break the eggs in the well and beat then pour in the orange extract, melted butter and whipping cream and stir until smooth. Add the slivered almonds and stir well.

Place the dough onto the earlier prepared cookie sheet then pat out a round loaf with your hands. Cut the dough into 8 wedges ensuring that there is some distance between them.

Bake until golden brown for 25 minutes then switch of the oven and let the scones stay in the oven for 10 to 15 more minutes.

Meanwhile, make the glaze by microwaving the powdered swerve, cream cheese and butter for around 30 seconds to 1 minute. Use a fork to mix well until you have a smooth glaze and the butter and cheese dissolve.

Drizzle the glaze over your scones and enjoy

Nutritional info per serving: Calories 217, Proteins 5g, Carbs 6g and Fats 20g

Ham & Cheese Pretzels

Prep time: 15 minutes

Cook time: 20 minutes

Total time: 35 minutes

Yields: 4 servings

Ingredients

6 oz Swiss cheese

6 oz ham

5 tablespoons of cream cheese

3 cups of shredded mozzarella cheese

3 large eggs, divided

1 teaspoon of onion powder

1 teaspoon of garlic powder

1 tablespoon of baking powder

2 cups of blanched almond flour

Pinch of coarse sea salt for topping

Keto Bread

Directions

Preheat your oven to 425 degrees F.

Prepare a rimmed baking sheet by lining with parchment paper.

Mix the onion powder, garlic powder, baking powder and almond flour in a medium mixing bowl and mix until well combined.

In a small bowl, crack one of the eggs and whisk with a fork – you will use this as the egg wash for the pretzels. The remaining eggs go in the dough.

Combine the cream cheese and mozzarella cheese in a large microwave-safe mixing bowl and microwave for 1 ½ minutes then remove and stir to combine.

Put back in the microwave for one more minute and mix again until well combined.

Add the almond flour mixture and the remaining eggs into the mixing bowl with the cheese mixture and mix until well incorporated.

Place the dough back in the microwave for 30 more seconds to soften if it gets unworkable and too stringy then continue mixing.

Keto Bread

Portion the dough into 6 equal pieces and roll each piece into a long thin piece such as a breadstick then fold each into a pretzel shape.

Use the egg wash to brush the top of each pretzel then add a piece of ham and Swiss cheese. Sprinkle the top with coarse sea salt and bake on the middle rack until golden brown for 12 to 14 minutes.

Nutritional info per serving: Calories 577, Protein 36g, Carbs 14g and Fat 44g

Keto Breadsticks

Prep time: 10 minutes

Cook time: 15 minutes

Total time: 25 minutes

Yields: 24 breadsticks

Ingredients

Breadstick base

1 teaspoon of baking powder

1 large egg

3 tablespoons of cream cheese

1 tablespoon of psyllium husk powder

¾ cup of almond flour

2 cups of shredded mozzarella cheese

For Italian style:

1 teaspoon of pepper

1 teaspoon of salt

2 tablespoons of Italian seasoning

Keto Bread

For extra cheesy:

¼ cup of parmesan cheese

3 ounces of cheddar cheese

1 teaspoon of onion powder

1 teaspoon of garlic powder

For cinnamon sugar:

2 tablespoons of cinnamon

6 tablespoons of swerve sweetener

3 tablespoons of butter

Directions

Preheat your oven to 400 degrees F.

Mix the cream cheese and egg until slightly combined then set aside.

Combine all dry ingredients: baking powder, psyllium husk and almond flour in a bowl.

In a microwave safe bowl microwave the mozzarella cheese in 20 second intervals stirring every time you remove from the microwave and continue to microwave until the cheese is sizzling.

Add the dry ingredients, cream cheese and eggs into the melted mozzarella and mix.

Knead the dough using your hands and set on a silpat once it's mixed. Press the dough until you have a baking sheet worth of dough.

Transfer the dough to a foil to cut using a pizza cutter. You should never use sharp objects and knives.

Cut the dough and season with the above ingredients.

Bake on the top rack until crisp for 13 to 15 minutes and serve warm.

Serving suggestion: serve the sweet bread sticks with cream cheese butter cream and the savory breadsticks with marinara

Nutritional info per serving

Italian style: Calories 238, Protein 12.8g, Carbs 2.6g and Fat 18.8g

Extra cheesy: Calories 314, Protein 18g, Carbs 3.6g and Fat 24.7g

Cinnamon sugar: Calories 291.7g, Protein 13g, Carbs 3.3g and Fat 24.3g

Keto Brioche Bread

Prep time: 5 minutes

Cook time: 30 minutes

Total time: 35 minutes

Yields: 2 servings

Ingredients

For the Brioche:

4 drops of liquid Stevia

½ teaspoon of lemon zest

½ teaspoon of vanilla bean paste

1 (28g) packet of natural grass-fed butter

1 large egg

¼ teaspoon of baking powder

1 (31g) packet of keto protein vanilla

Blueberry sauce:

½ teaspoon of pure vanilla extract

1 teaspoon of fresh lemon juice

Keto Bread

1 pinch of salt

1 (1g) packet of Stevia/erythritol blend

2/3 cup of frozen blueberries

Other (optional)

Swerve confectioners for garnish

Directions

Preheat your oven to 350 degrees F.

Prepare a 6 oz ramekin by greasing the inside with coconut oil or butter.

In a medium bowl, whisk together all ingredients then pour them into the ramekin.

Bake for about 25-30 minutes until the brioche is golden and puffed and a toothpick comes out clean when inserted into the brioche.

Meanwhile make the blueberry sauce by placing the blueberries, salt and Stevia in a microwave safe bowl. Microwave for 6 minutes stopping half way through to stir.

Stir in the vanilla and lemon juice once out of the microwave (you can also make the sauce on a stovetop).

Top the brioche with the blueberry sauce and serve. You can also dust the top with swerve confectioners if desired.

Nutritional info per serving: Calories 178, Protein 3g, Carbs 8g and Fat 15g

Low Carb Garlic Bread

Prep time: 5 minutes

Cook time: 25 minutes

Total time: 30 minutes

Yields: 4 servings

Ingredients

1 tablespoon of freshly grated Parmesan

1 tablespoon of freshly chopped parsley

1 clove of garlic, minced

1 tablespoon of butter, melted

1 large egg

1 teaspoon of baking powder

1 tablespoon of garlic powder

2 tablespoons of cream cheese

1/2 cup of finely ground almond flour

1 cup of shredded mozzarella

Kosher salt

Keto Bread

Marinara, warmed, for serving

Directions

Preheat your oven to 400 degrees F.

Line a baking sheet with parchment paper.

In a medium microwave safe bowl, add the baking powder, garlic powder, a large pinch of salt, cream cheese, almond flour and mozzarella cheese. Microwave for about 1 minute on high until the cheeses melts. Stir in the egg.

Place the dough onto the prepared baking sheet and shape it into a ½" thick oval.

Mix the melted butter with parmesan, parsley and garlic in a small bowl. Brush the mixture on top of the bread.

Bake for 15 to 17 minutes until golden. Slice and serve warm with marinara sauce.

Nutritional info per serving: Calories 117, Protein 11.2g, Carbs 4.6g and Fat 6.32g

Sweet Challah Bread

Prep time: 10 minutes

Cook time: 45 minutes

Total time: 55 minutes

Yields: 22 servings

Ingredients

¼ cup of dried cranberries

½ lemon zest

1 teaspoon of xanthan gum

2 ½ teaspoons of baking powder

1/3 teaspoon of baking soda

½ teaspoon of salt

2/3 cup of vanilla protein

1 cup of unflavored protein

50g of oil

60g of heavy cream

60g of butter

Keto Bread

345g of cream cheese

50g of Sukrin plus

4 eggs

Directions

Preheat your oven to 320 degrees F (160 C).

Mix the eggs until soft peaks for, and then add in then add in the sugar substitute and mix once more.

Add the cream cheese and the remaining liquid ingredients and mix again.

Add in all the dry ingredients once the mixture is properly mixed and mix.

Use a mixer to combine the fresh lemon zest and the cranberries then hand mix it gently into the dough.

Place the dough on a silicone baking pan according to your desired shape and bake for 45 minutes.

Nutritional info per serving: Calories 158, Protein 9g, Carbs 2g and Fat 13g

Cheesy Breadsticks

Prep time: 10 minutes

Cook time: 15 minutes

Total time: 25 minutes

Yields: 8 servings

Ingredients

For the breadsticks

½ cup of parmesan cheese, shredded

1 1/3 cups of mozzarella cheese, shredded

½ teaspoon of garlic powder

1 teaspoon of Italian seasoning

¼ teaspoon of baking powder

½ teaspoon of salt

4 eggs

1 oz of cream cheese, softened

1/3 cup of coconut flour

4 ½ tablespoons of butter (melted and cooled)

Keto Bread

For the top

12 teaspoons of Italian seasoning

¼ cup of parmesan cheese, shredded

2 cups of mozzarella cheese, shredded

Directions

Preheat your oven to 400 degrees F.

Prepare a 11*7 baking pan by greasing it.

Combine the cream cheese, salt, eggs and melted butter then mix.

Add the spices, baking powder and coconut flour to the butter mixture and stir until combined then stir in the parmesan and mozzarella.

Transfer the batter to a casserole dish then top with the additional Italian spices, parmesan cheese and mozzarella.

Bake until the breadsticks are done for 15 minutes. Halfway through baking, use a pizza cutter to create individual breadsticks.

Transfer the pan to the top rack of your oven and broil until the cheese is bubbly and brown for around 1-2 minutes

Keto Bread

Serve with keto friendly marinara sauce,

Nutritional info per serving: Calories 299, Proteins 17g, Carbs 4g and Fats 23g

Keto Scones

Prep time: 10 minutes

Cook time: 40 minutes

Total time: 50 minutes

Yields: 8 servings

Ingredients

2/3 cup of coarsely chopped pecans

2 teaspoons of maple extract

2 ½ tablespoons of cold butter (chopped into small pieces)

1 large egg

½ cup of heavy cream

1 tablespoon of baking powder

½ teaspoon of salt

2 tablespoons of collagen

¼ cup of sweetener

½ cup of coconut flour

1 1/2 cups of almond flour

Keto Bread

For maple glaze:

2 teaspoons of water

1 tablespoon of heavy cream

1 teaspoon of maple extract

½ cup of powdered erythritol

Directions

Preheat your oven to 350 degrees F.

Prepare your baking sheet by lining with parchment paper.

Add the dry ingredients to your food processor and pulse until well combined. Add in extract, butter, egg and the cream then pulse until you form crumbs. Add in the pecans and process until the dough forms a ball. This takes around 1 to 2 minutes.

Place the dough onto the prepared baking sheet and press to form a circle then cut into 8 wedges. Spread them out to leave at least half an inch between them.

Bake until golden and firm for 40 minutes. Cover the scones with foil if they begin to get dark – check them after 15 to 20 minutes. Cool completely.

Prepare the maple glaze by combining all glaze ingredients then spread on your cooled scones. Enjoy

Nutritional info per serving: Calories 302, Protein 7g, Carbs 11g and Fat 27g

Conclusion

Thank you for purchasing the book and taking the time to read it.

Sticking with the ketogenic diet was challenging for me especially since you cannot eat bread. However, those recipes have made it easier to follow the keto diet and I hope they do the same for you.

All the best in your quest for a healthier YOU.

Finally, I would like to ask you for a favor. Can you please leave a review for this book? I will greatly appreciate that.

Thank you and Good Luck!

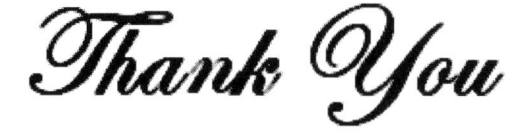

Thank You

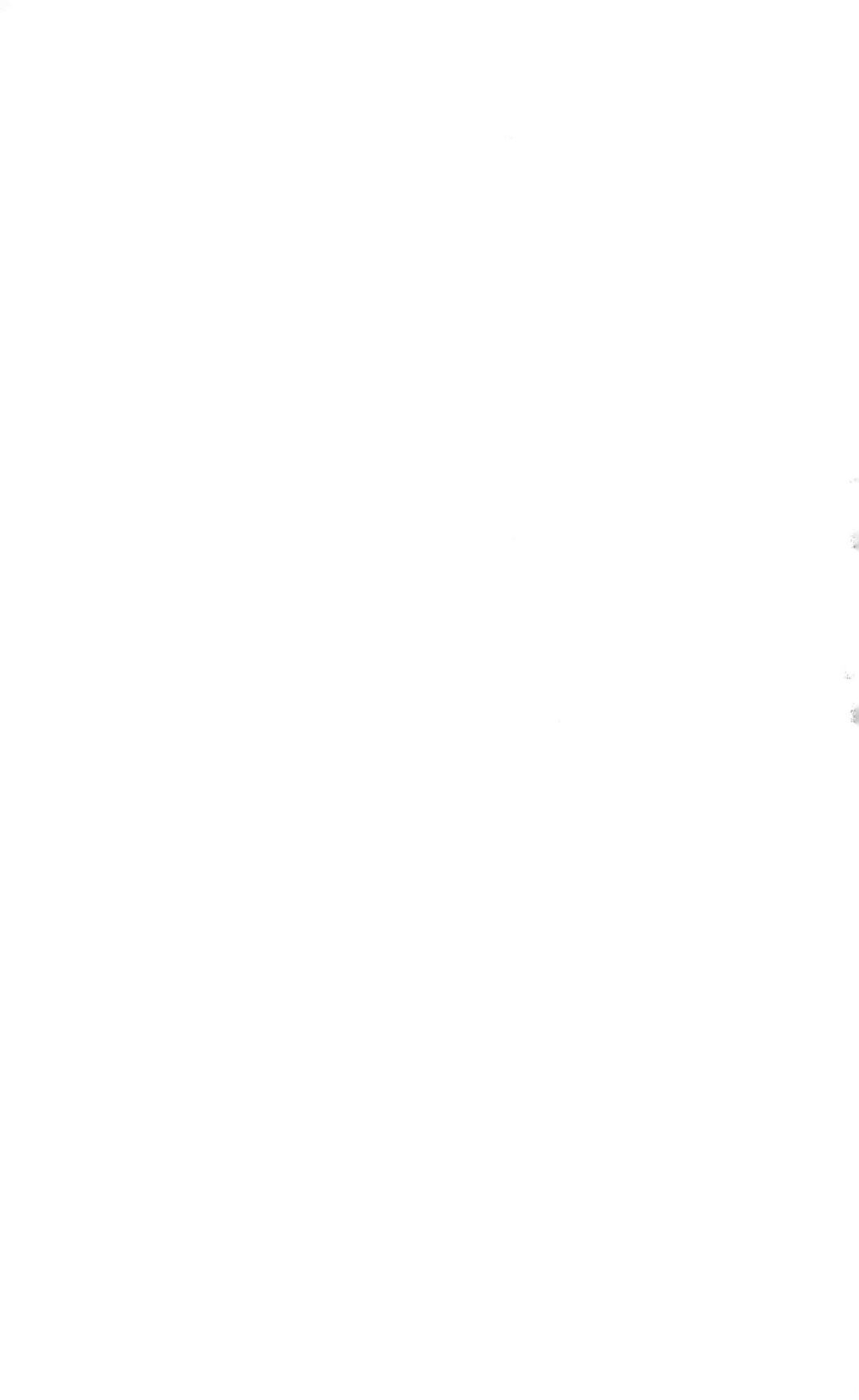

Printed in Great Britain
by Amazon